7 MINUTE FITNESS FIX

THE GUIDE TO A TOTAL TRANSFORMATION

NO GYM WEIGHTS EQUIPMENT

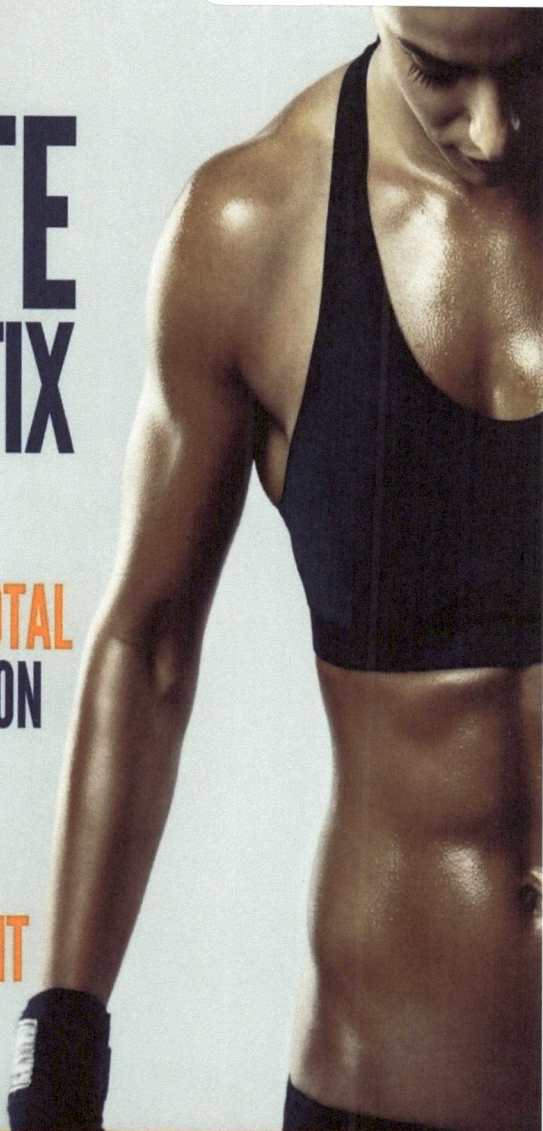

TISHA MEADS

CERTIFIED PERSONAL TRAINER

7 Minute Fitness Fix

Copyright 2017 by LaTisha Meads

Meal Plans & Smoothie Recipes prepared by:
Dr. Victoria Stroman, Health Coach, Holistic Essentials, LLC
www.naturalself.net | vchiro09@gmail.com

Cover Design by: Otis Spears

7 Minute Fitness Fix

Foreword

As Director of Education of the National Personal Training Institute of Houston my passion has been helping develop, coach, mentor, and teach students to become personal trainers, strength coaches, and wellness professionals. Tisha entered the personal training program in July of 2014, and although reserved as a new student her passion for helping others quickly began to blossom along with her distinctive training style. Right from the start she had a mission to make fitness and wellness a fun filled experience that is not only effective but convenient. She has worked tirelessly on improving herself, her training abilities, and her growth as a coach. Tisha is not just a certified personal trainer; she is a qualified personal trainer who is passionate on achieving results and motivating others. Her book is designed to give the reader an easy, fun, and effective workout regimen and provide guidance on improving overall health and wellness. Many students have graduated from the personal training program; however, Tisha has proven herself time and time again to be one of the more persistent and dedicated trainers, delivering high quality services to all her clients. As an educator, it makes me proud to have made such a strong impact on Tisha's drive and passion. With her continued success, I will continuously provide my support and guidance whenever she should need, and look forward to her bright future in this industry.

- David Boettcher
  Director of Education
  National Personal Training Institute of Houston

The pages you are about to dive into as you enhance your health & wellness could not make me prouder as the author's former instructor. Over the course of six months, Tisha was consistently one of our top students, taking what was taught to her and always expanding on the finer details. Perhaps her strongest characteristic is her hunger to continuously improve and be a leader in the field of exercise and nutrition. That desire is demonstrated by the countless hours that went into the production of this book. Tisha's knowledge and experience shines bright as she guides you down the correct path toward optimal workouts and nutritional advice.

- Jay Sutaria
  Owner, ST&F LLC
  Former Instructor - National Personal Training Institute

Overview

7 Minute Fitness Fix is for those who want to maintain a "fit" lifestyle. Whether you are a beginner, intermediate, or advanced/athletic trainee, you will find that these routines are: fun, interesting, challenging, and will get you to the next level you are looking for. *7 Minute Fitness Fix* provides an easy start solution for those who don't know where to start and/or just looking for a change in routine. Fitness is not just exercising daily, it includes a healthy and balanced diet. I have included recipes and meal plans that will aid you in reaching your fitness goals.

If you don't like the gym, NO PROBLEM! These routines can be done at the park or in home. Don't worry about not knowing the names of different exercises because illustrations of the exercises are included. The routines are numbered by the level. Beginners would start with 1, intermediates are 2, and advance trainees are 3. This doesn't limit you from putting them together. Once you have become good at your level, mix and match different levels together for another challenge.

To get the best results, we want, here's how we do it:
1. Begin our workout with a positive attitude, focusing on our results.
2. Find an accountability partner, someone to help us.
3. Workout at least 3 times per week, make the time to fit it in.
4. Perform each exercise correctly, let's not cheat ourselves.
5. DO NOT GIVE UP, push through and FINISH the workout!
6. Eat healthy! Follow the recipes in this book.

Show off your achievements and inspire others! Send your BEFORE & AFTER pictures to the email below. We will feature you on our website and other media outlets.

CONTACT INFO:

Email: info@cmofit.com

Website: www.cmofit.com

Phone: 713-494-2815

Facebook, YouTube: C'MOfitness or @CMOfitness

Instagram, Twitter, Periscope: @CMO_fitness

Snapchat: @chantzes

Choosing Your Workout

Don't focus on how much time you are going to work out, take it ONE MINUTE AT A TIME! The idea is… you are going to split your workout into *7 Minute* segments, doing each exercise for 1 minute. There are several options when choosing your workout. Your choice will be based on the area of your body you want to workout. For example, if you want to focus on legs, you would do one or more of the lower body routines; if you want to target your arms and/or chest, you would do one or more of the upper body routines; if you want to work on your whole body, you would do one or more of the full bodies or pick any combonation of the routines; and so on. GET TO IT!

suggested levels:
beginners, half workout intermediate/advanced/athlete, full workout

FULL WORKOUT = 50 – 90 minutes

- Warm-up by stretching, cardio, or 1 round of one of the full body routines
- Perform routine for 5 – 8 rounds
- Cool down by stretching or foam rolling

(warm-up & cool down should last 5 – 10 minutes)

REST PERIODS:

a) 2 – 3 minutes after each round

b) 30 seconds between each exercise & 1 – 2 minutes between each round

HALF WORKOUT = 25 – 40 minutes

- Warm-up
- Perform routine 3 – 4 rounds
- Cool down
- Rest periods are the same

Routines

Visit my YouTube page for video of each exercise.
Search "7 Minute Book The Video" or go to
www.youtube.com/cmofitness

Full Body 1

modified jacks

1. Jumping Jacks
- to modify, lift one leg up at a time

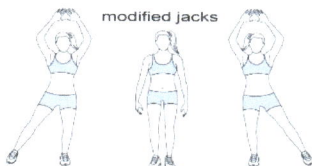

2. Front Kicks
- keep your core tight

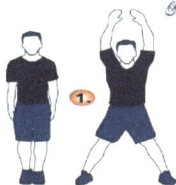

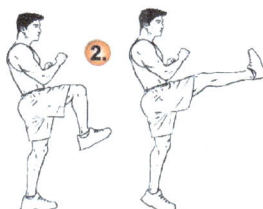

3. Side Kicks
- keep your core tight

4. Low (fore arm) Plank
- be sure to keep core tight and back straight, no arching

5. Squats
- keep your core tight, don't lean over or bend your back, keep knees out, and sit back as if you were sitting in a chair

6. Modified Mountain Climbers
- instead of switching both feet at the same time, step one foot out and back in at a time

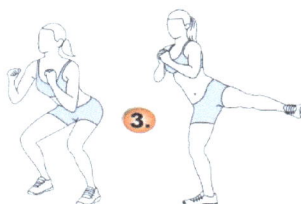

7. Bird Dogs
- be sure to keep back straight

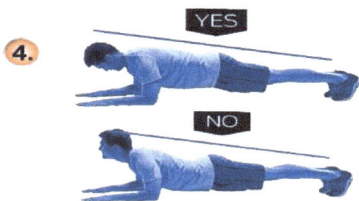

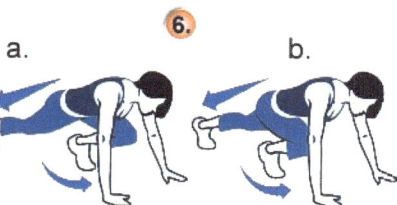

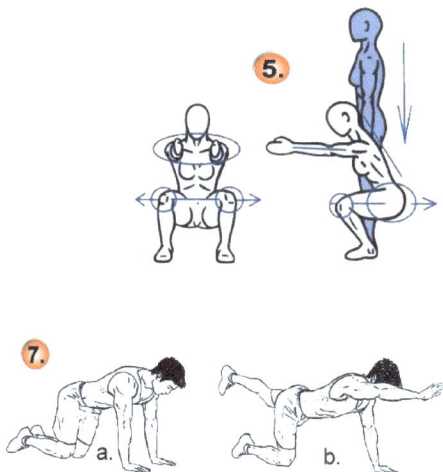

YES

NO

a. b.

a. b.

Full Body 2

1. 4 Way Kicks
- kick both legs to the front, then both legs to each side, putting front and side kicks together (previous page)

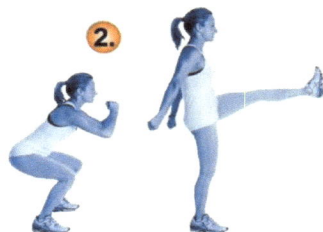

2. Squat to Front Kick
- keep your core tight, don't lean over or bend your back

3. Cross Jumping Jacks
- keep core tight

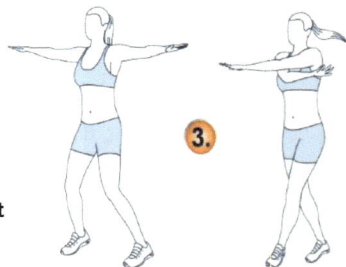

4. High Plank
- be sure to keep your core tight and back straight

5. Floor Taps
- as you bend over keep core tight to not pull from your lower back

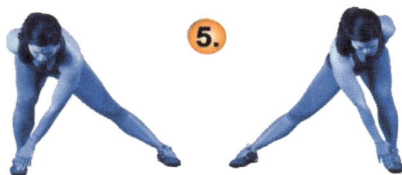

6. Squat Hold & Punch
- squeeze your butt while holding squat

7. Modified Burpee
- instead of hopping out with both feet at once, step one foot out and in at a time

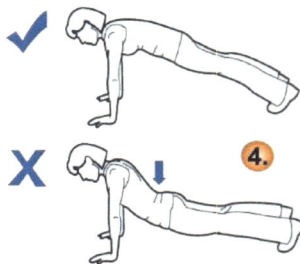

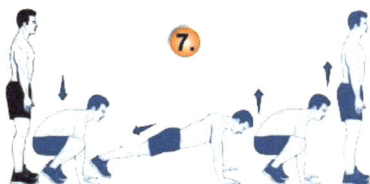

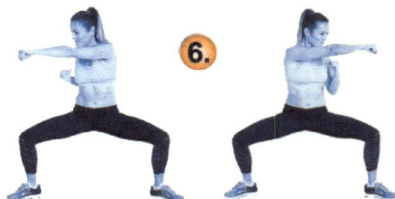

Full Body 3

1. Burpees
 - when popping back into a squat, bring
   your feet wide close to your hands,
   not in right under chest

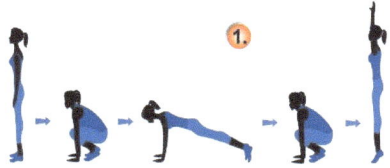

2. Low Plank Rock
 - keep your core tight as you rock

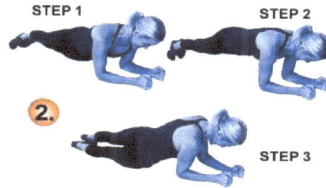

3. Knee Ups w/ Bounce
 - don't bend over and keep core tight

4. Plank Push-up
 - be sure to keep core tight

5. Russian Twists
 - keep back straight, no arching

6. Squat Jacks
 - stay low while performing
   and core tight

7. Mountain Climbers
 - keep your core tight, no piking

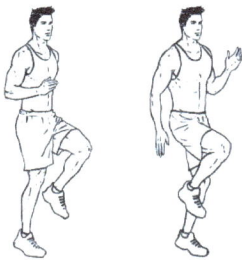

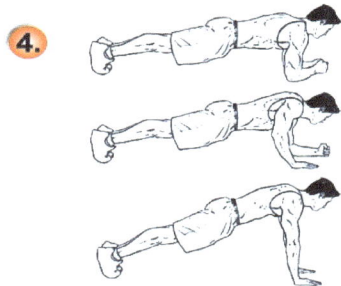

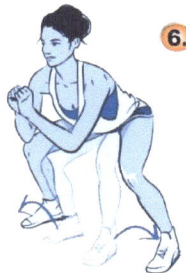

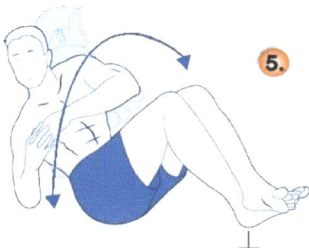

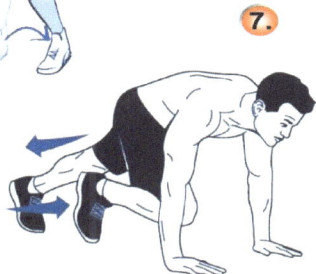

STEP 1   STEP 2   STEP 3

Upper Body

Upper Body 1

1. High Plank
  - be sure to keep your core tight
    and back straight

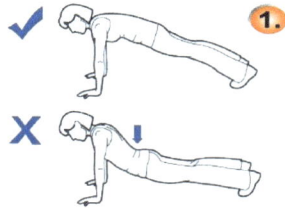

2. Standing Side Crunch
  - you want to keep your core tight, don't
    bend too far over, connect elbow with
    knee in the middle

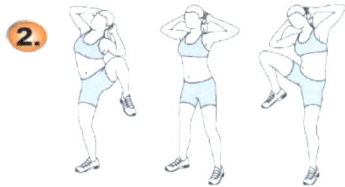

3. Low (fore arm) Plank
  - be sure to keep core tight and
    back straight, no arching

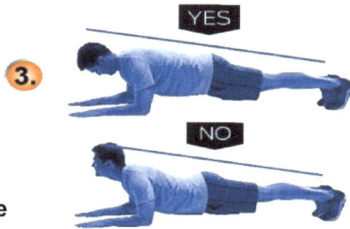

4. High Plank w/ Shoulder Tap
  - keep core tight and back straight,
    no dipping or arching

5. Straight Leg Sit-ups
  - be sure to keep core tight, back
    straight and no arching

6. Modified Mtn. Climbers
  - instead of switching both feet at the
    same time, step one foot out and
    back in at a time

7. Walkouts
  - in standing position, walkout with hands
    then walk hands back to feet, return to
    standing position and repeat

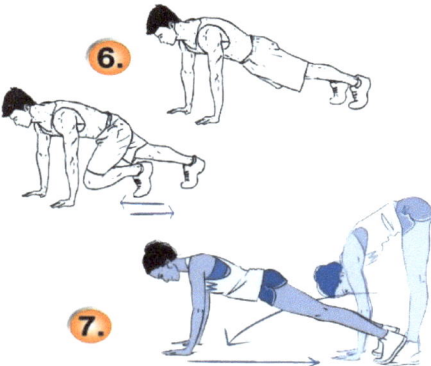

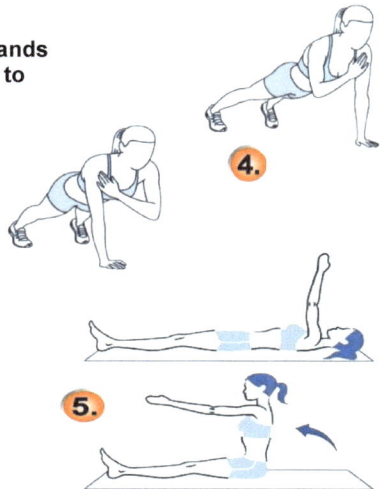

Upper Body 2

1.

1. Plank & Reach Through
- be sure to keep core tight

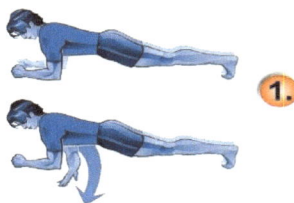

2. Modified V-sit Ins
- keep back straight using a tight core to raise upper body

2.

3. Modified Plank Jacks
- instead of hopping both feet out at the same time, step one foot to the side and back in at a time

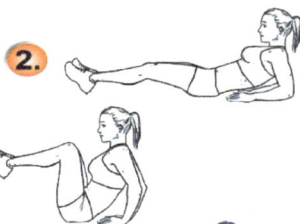

4. Push-ups
- keep core tight and back straight, no dipping or arching

3.

5. Ankle Taps
- have your feet spaced good enough so you can feel it in your obliques

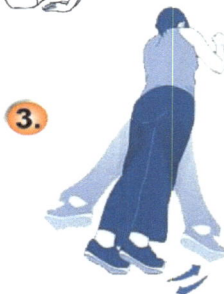

6. Mountain Climbers
- as you switch your feet back and forth keep your core tight, no piking butt

7. High Plank Rock
- this is like low plank rocks. (FB3) keep your core tight as you rock

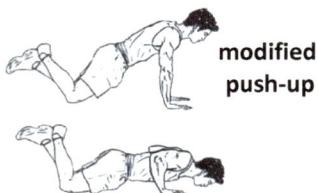

modified push-up

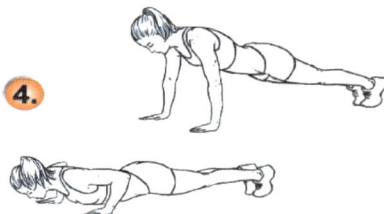

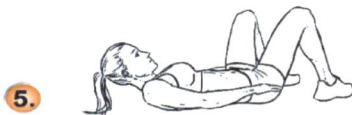

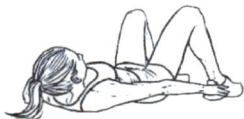

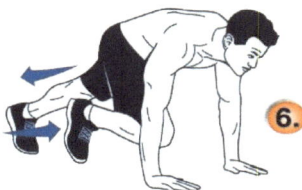

4.

5.

6.

Upper Body 3

1. Inchworms
- in standing position, walkout with hands then walk feet to hands, and repeat

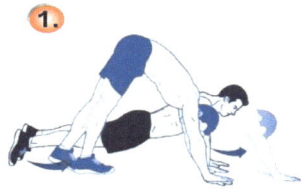

2. X's & O's
- lie back with hands & feet spread wide, then squeeze your stomach to come up bringing hands & legs into your chest like a ball, keep back straight no arching

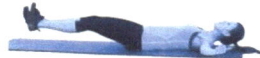

3. Plank Push-ups
- keep core tight and back straight, no dipping or arching

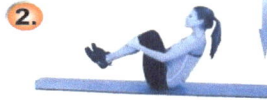

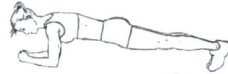

4. V-ups
- keep core tight and back straight, no arching

5. Cross Mtn. Climbers
- twist your core while bringing your knee in and over to opposite arm don't pike your butt, keep core tight

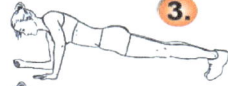

6. Plank Jacks
- be sure to keep core tight

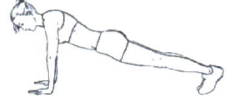

7. Spiderman Push-ups
- keep your core tight and back straight

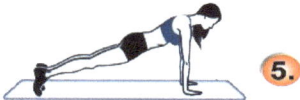

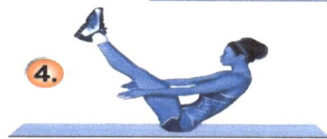

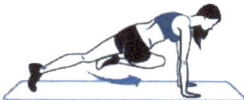

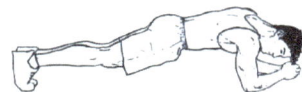

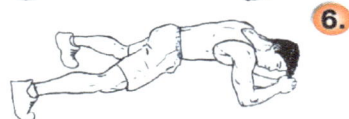

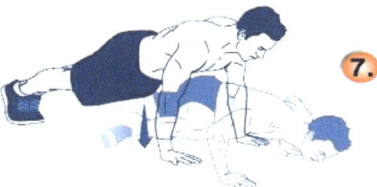

Core

Core 1

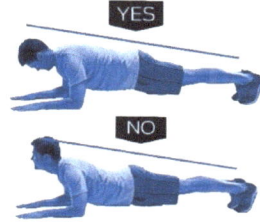

1. Low (fore arm) Plank
- keep your core tight, no arching or dipping

2. Bird Dog
- donkey kick one leg back and reach the opposite hand out in front at the same time, keep your core tight

3. Side Plank
- keep your core tight, to modify drop to one or both knees

4. High Plank
- be sure to keep core tight and back straight

5. Knees to Chest
- place hands under your lower back if needed for more support

6. Modified Mtn. Climbers
- instead of switching both feet at the same time, step one foot out and back in at a time

7. Straight Leg Sit-ups
- be sure to keep core tight, back straight and no arching

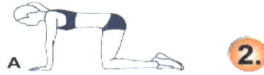

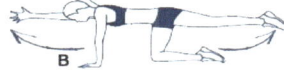

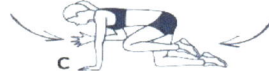

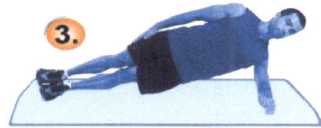

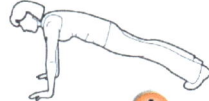

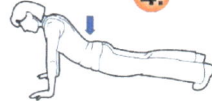

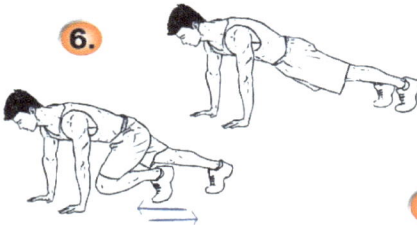

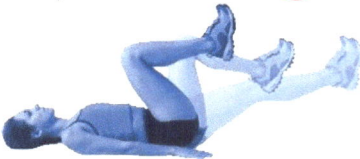

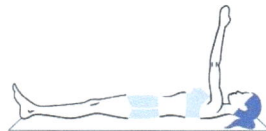

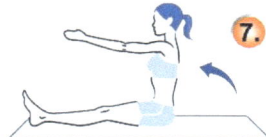

Core 2

1. Cross Body Knee Jabs
- you want to keep your core tight, don't bend too far over, connect elbow with knee in the middle

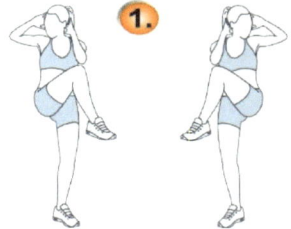

2. Low Plank Rocks
- keep your core tight as you rock

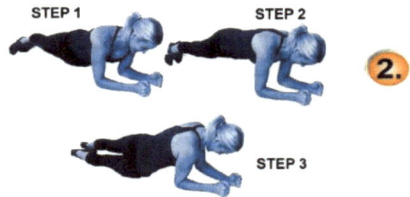

3. Side Plank Drop
- keep your core tight

4. High Plank Bird Dog
- be sure to keep core tight

5. Low Plank Pike
- keep your core tight

6. High Plank Reach
- be sure to keep core tight, back straight and no arching

7. Mountain Climbers
- keep your core tight, no piking

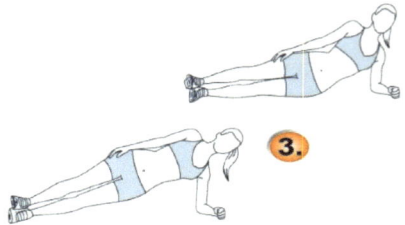

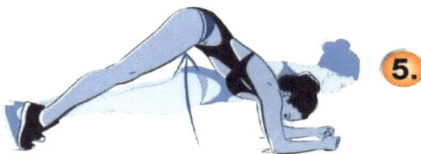

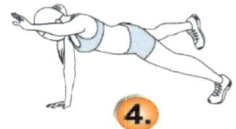

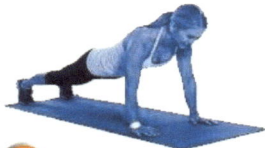

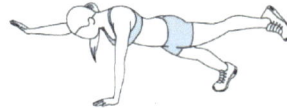

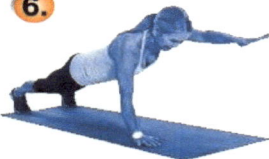

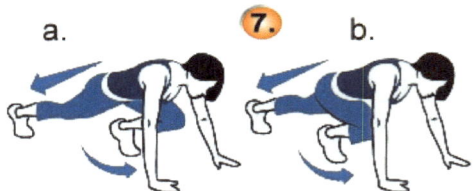

STEP 1   STEP 2

STEP 3

a.   b.

Core 3

1. Russian Twists
   - be sure to keep core tight, back straight and no arching

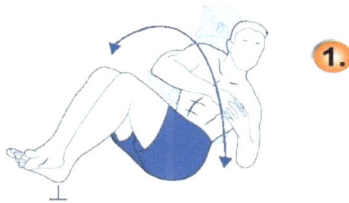

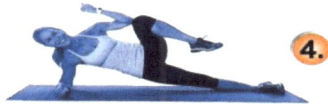

2. Plank Jacks
   - keep core tight

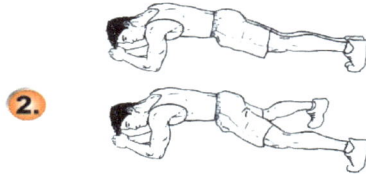

3. Crab Toe Touch
   - keep back straight as possible and core tight

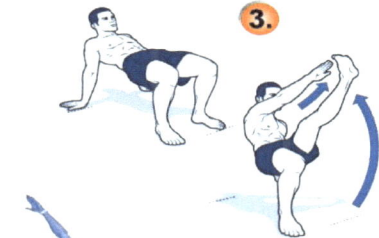

4. Side Plank Crunch
   - to modify drop to one knee, keep your core tight

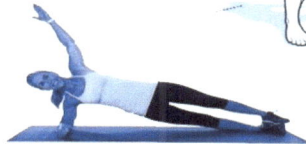

5. Alternate Toe Touch
   - be sure to keep core tight, back straight and no arching

6. X's & O's
   - keep back straight, no arching

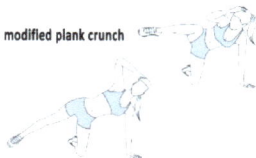

7. V-ups
   - no arching when performing

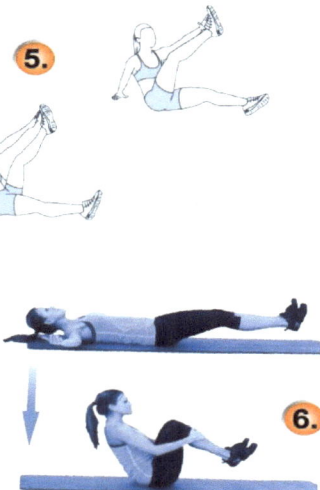

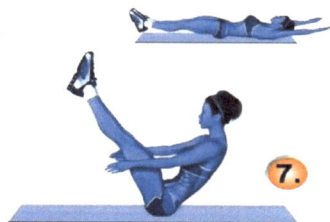

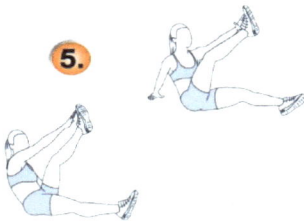

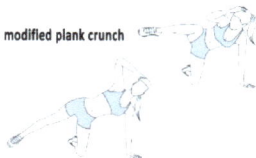

modified plank crunch

Lower
Body

Lower Body 1

1. Side to Side Hops
   - pick a line or something to hop over

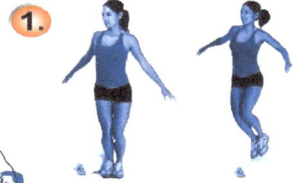

2. Reverse Lunge
   - keep weight front leg dominate, don't put pressure on back knee

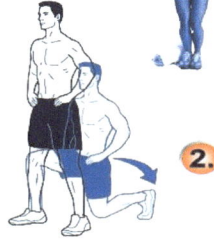

3. Lying Side Leg Raise
   - lie on your side in a straight position

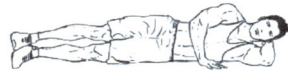

4. Squats
   - keep your core tight, don't lean over or bend your back, keep knees out, and sit back as if you were sitting in a chair

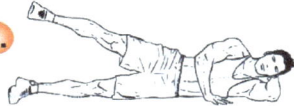

5. Knee Ups w/ Bounce
   - don't bend over and keep core tight

6. Hip Lifts (thrusts)
   - squeeze your butt as you lift your hips

7. Low Plank w/ Leg Raise
   - be sure to keep core tight

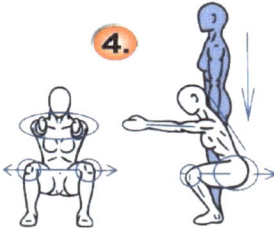

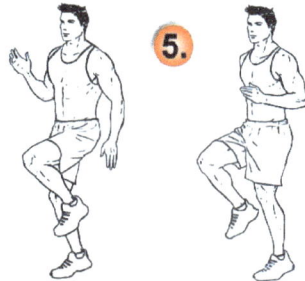

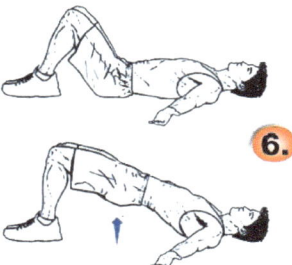

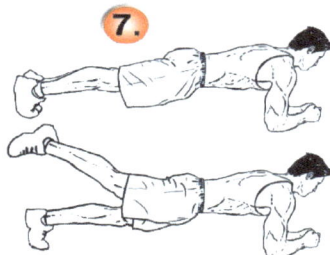

Lower Body 2

1. Plie Squats
   - in a slightly wide squat stance,
     turn feet out 45 degrees, don't let
     knees go pass your toes

2. Skaters
   - as you go to the side keep butt tight

3. Star Jumps
   - when landing bend your knees a little
     to relieve some of the pressure on the joint

4. Side Lunge
   - as you lunge to the side toot butt
     back as if you were sitting in a chair

5. Side Hop w/ Floor Tap
   - keep your core tight

6. Squat to Side Leg Lift
   - keep your core tight, don't lean over
     or bend your back

7. Reverse Lunge to Front Kick
   - keep weight front leg dominate, don't
     put pressure on back knee

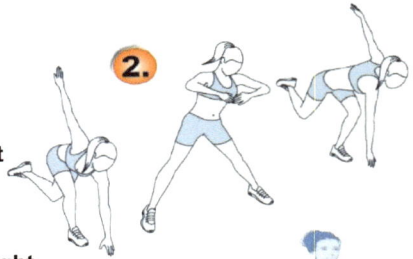
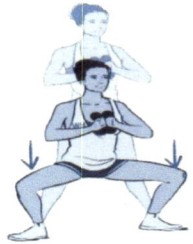
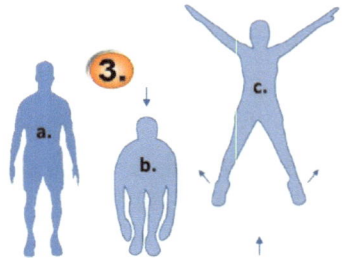
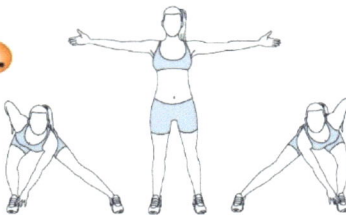
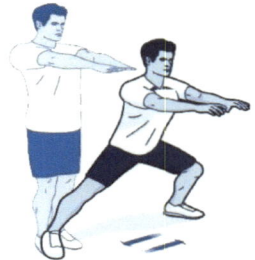
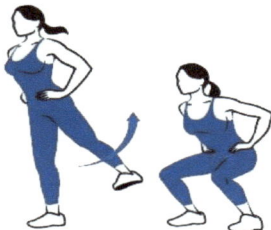
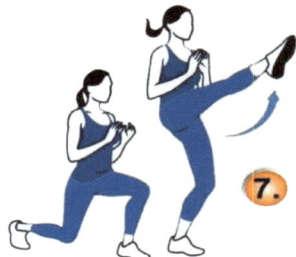

Lower Body 3

1. T-jacks
- keep core tight

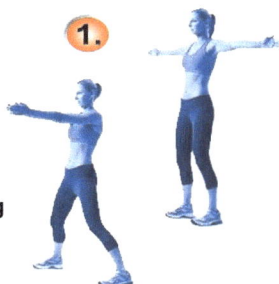

2. Squat Jacks
- stay low while performing and core tight

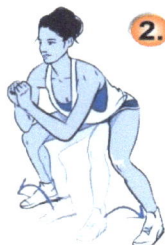

3. Jump Lunge
- keep weight front leg dominate, don't put pressure on back knee

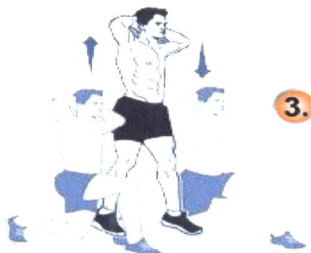

4. Single Leg Hip Thrust
- squeeze your butt as you lift your hips

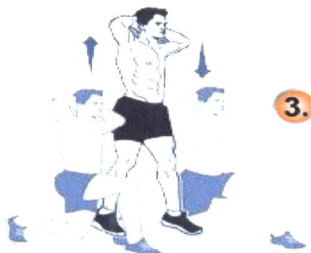

5. Tuck Jumps
- to modify, tuck one foot at at time under your butt

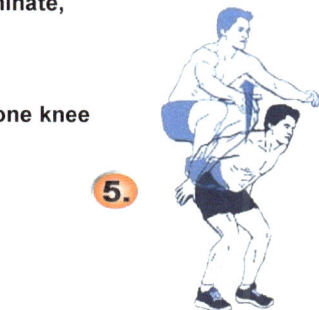

6. Reverse Lunge to Knee Up
- bring leg back into a lunge, then bring that same leg back up, raising knee up while using other leg to hop up, keep weight front leg dominate, don't put pressure on back knee

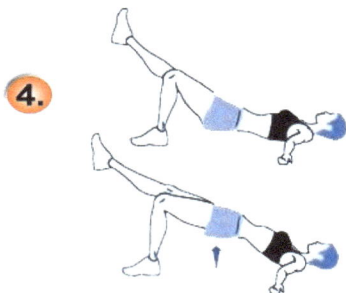

7. Side Plank w/ Side Leg Raise
- keep your core tight, to modify drop to one knee

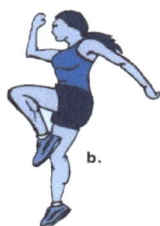

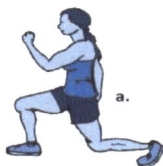

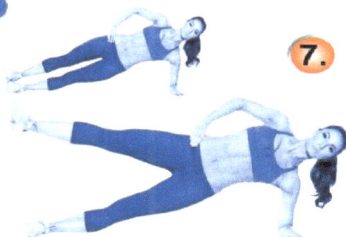

Smoothie Recipes

Prepared by Dr. Victoria Stroman, Health Coach
Holistic Essentials, LLC

Smoothie 1

Mango Banana SuperFood Smoothie Bowl

1.5 cup milk (Almond milk)

½ Avocado

1 scoop of protein

¼ Mango pulp (frozen Goya)

1-1.5 banana (frozen)

1 teaspoon Grind flax seed

Blend into a thick smoothie then add your toppings:
Golgi berries, Mulberries, nuts, pumpkin seeds or any
other fruit you would like to put on top. i.e. blueberries

Serving Size:
- Snack = ¾ cup (6 oz.)
- Meal Replacement = 1 ½ - 2 cups (12 – 16 oz.)
  with a cup of water

Digestive Smoothie

1.5 cup of milk (Almond Milk)

1/3 cup frozen Blueberries

2 tablespoon Chia seeds

1 Frozen Banana

* Use raw honey if you need sweeter

First thing in the morning, drink 4-8 ounces warm water with pink Himalayan sea salt to get bowels moving. Chia seeds are very good for the digestive system; helps stay hydrated longer, stay full longer, and good for the heart/brain function. Chia Seeds are loaded with vitamins and minerals.

Serving Size:
- Snack = 1 – 1 ¼ cup (8 – 10 oz.)
- Meal Replacement = 1 ½ - 2 cups (12 – 16 oz.)

Smoothie 3

Green Smoothie

1.5 cup Milk or Apple Juice (Cold Pressed)
1 teaspoon Almond Butter or Peanut Butter
4 Pitted Dates
Handful Kale or Spinach
¼ cup frozen raspberries
1.5 frozen Banana
1 Scoop of protein powder
Hint of Cinnamon

OR

1.5 cup Apple Juice (Cold Pressed)
½ cup Spinach or kale
2 frozen Banana
Protein Powder
1 tablespoon of coconut oil
2 tablespoons of raw hempseed (optional)

Benefit of hempseed: Great for cardiovascular system, provides protein, hormonal balance, and aid in digestion as well due to its fiber content. Raw hempseeds are loaded with minerals.

* Note- Buy bananas, peel then freeze in a Ziploc bag.

Serving Size:
- Snack = 1 – 1 ¼ cup (8 – 10 oz.)
- Meal Replacement = 1 ½ - 2 cups (12 – 16 oz.)

Meal Plans

Prepared by Dr. Victoria Stroman, Health Coach
Holistic Essentials, LLC

With these meal plans you can go about it 1 of 2 ways:

1. Pick the lunch or the dinner meal to cook and eat it for both lunch and dinner.

2. Cook a small portion of both, the lunch & the dinner meal, and eat as is, one for lunch and the other for dinner.

Portions:
Suggested by Tisha Meads, CPT
(Tisha is not a nutritionist, these portions are
only suggestions given through her professional experience.
Feel free to use these meals with the suggested portions from
your doctor or preferred nutritionist.)

Meal Plan 1

Breakfast: before 10am
8 – 16 oz. of room temperature water first thing upon waking up. *(8oz when you first wake up and 8 oz. after you finished getting dressed.)*

21 oz. Green Smoothie *(use almond butter for protein)*
Consisting 1 cup green veggies and 1/2 cup green fruit made with unsweetened Almond milk *(silk or almond breeze)*

Lunch: before 2pm
Meat: Salmon 3 oz.

Starch/Carbs: Baked sweet potato ½ of medium OR 1 small
OR
Wild rice ½ cup

Vegetable: Asparagus 1 cup

Dinner: before 7pm
Meat & Starch/Carbs: Rice Pasta OR Spaghetti Squash ½ cup with Meat sauce (½ cup) *(use lean beef 97% lean & 3% fat or ground turkey for the meat sauce)*

Vegetables & Fruit: Green Salad (small bowl/cereal sized bowl) & 1 cup Fresh Fruit

2 Snacks: 1 in between breakfast and lunch & 1 in between lunch and dinner.
1 bottle water or if you use reusable bottle at least 2 cups 16 oz.

WITH

1 Granola bar oats & honey OR 1 Trail Mix bar fruit & nuts OR 1 Kellogg's NutriGrain Bar

OR

1 whole fruit (orange, apple, banana, or pear…etc.)

* If you don't like the suggested snacks, keep the water, but choose a healthy snack that works for you.

** Vegetarians can substitute beans for meats or a veggie meat alternative

*** Drinks: stay away from sugary drinks such as soda and juices with lots of sugar. Intake at least 64oz of water per day.

Meal Plan 2

Breakfast: before 10am
8 – 16 oz. of room temperature water first thing upon waking up. *(8oz when you first wake up and 8 oz. after you finished getting dressed.)*

2 poached eggs, 1 slice of multigrain toast, warm spinach salad

Lunch: before 2pm
Meat: baked Chicken breast 3 oz.

Starch/Carbs: roasted red potatoes 2/3 cup

Vegetable: Spinach OR Broccoli 1 cup

Dinner: before 7pm
Meat: Grilled chicken breast 3oz

Vegetables & Fruit: 2/3 cup mixed vegetables & 1 cup cucumber and tomato salad

2 Snacks: 1 in between breakfast and lunch & 1 in between lunch and dinner.
1 bottle water or if you use reusable bottle at least 2 cups (16 oz.)

WITH

½ cup of Trail Mix fruit & nuts OR 1 small bag of the 100 calorie snacks

OR

1 whole fruit (mango, (½ cup) berries, (½ cup) cantaloupe…etc)

* If you don't like the suggested snacks, keep the water, but choose a healthy snack that works for you.

** Vegetarians can substitute beans for meats or a veggie meat alternative

*** Drinks: stay away from sugary drinks such as soda and juices with lots of sugar. Intake at least 64oz of water per day.

Meal Plan 3

Breakfast: before 10am
8 – 16 oz. of room temperature water first thing upon waking up. *(8oz when you first wake up and 8 oz. after you finished getting dressed.)*

21 oz. smoothie made with Quinoa flakes, Fresh Fruit, & Natural juice

Lunch: before 2pm
Meat: Beef (leanest) medium rare 3 oz.

Starch/Carbs: Brown rice ½ cup

Vegetable: Steam kale 1 cup

Dinner: before 7pm
Meat: Salmon 3oz

Vegetables & Starch/Carbs: 1 cup zucchini & yellow squash, 1 cup spinach w/ mushroom

2 Snacks: 1 in between breakfast and lunch & 1 in between lunch and dinner.
1 bottle water or if you use reusable bottle at least 2 cups (16 oz.)

WITH

½ cup of Trail Mix fruit & nuts OR 12 oz. fruit smoothie

OR

1 whole fruit (plum, (½ cup) grapes, peach etc)

* If you don't like the suggested snacks, keep the water, but choose a healthy snack that works for you.

** Vegetarians can substitute beans for meats or a veggie meat alternative

*** Drinks: stay away from sugary drinks such as soda and juices with lots of sugar.
Intake at least 64oz of water per day.

Notes

Here is where we keep track of our progression. We are going to start with listing our goals: short term and long term, 45 day goal, and 90 day goal. Next, write down where we are now. Then, check-in in 45 days by jotting down our accomplishments. Followed by, a 90 day check-in where we jot down our accomplishments again, as well as, make new goals, if necessary, or readjustments to continue working on our originals goals.

Things, we can track:
Weight, body measurements, body fat, endurance (how long you were able to last without stopping), maximum reps/weight lifted…etc.

Notes

Notes

Notes

Thank You

First, I would like to thank YOU for allowing me to help you improve your health & fitness by your investment in this manual. If it wasn't for people like you I wouldn't have a job to do. Next, thank you to all of my supporters who helped put this together: Victoria Stroman for the great recipes and David Boettcher & Jay Sutaria for writing genuine words in their foreword, as well as being great and amazing instructors that helped/helps guide me to be a better trainer. Onward, to all my clients who trust in me enough to help get them the incredible results they desire. If it weren't for you I wouldn't have living proof or anyone to brag about! Last, but never least, my father Zack Meads IV and my spiritual parents RC & Lisa Blakes for always believing, reassuring, and encouraging me. To my sister Johna Hill thank you for always being in my corner. You're always willing to be anything I need, from: editing, reviewing, help designing, ready to say yes or no go, or whatever it is advice on. So, THANK YOU!

I love you all and thank you again for helping produce this life changing manual!

GET TISHA OUT TO YOUR NEXT EVENT!

- HEALTH & FITNESS
  - CAREER DAY
  - RETREATS
- WOMEN'S EMPOWERMENT
  - KID'S FITNESS
    ETC.

CONTACT INFO:

Email: info@cmofit.com

Website: www.cmofit.com

Phone: 713-494-2815

Facebook, YouTube: C'MOfitness or

@CMOfitness

Instagram, Twitter, Periscope: @CMO_fitness

Snapchat: @chantzes

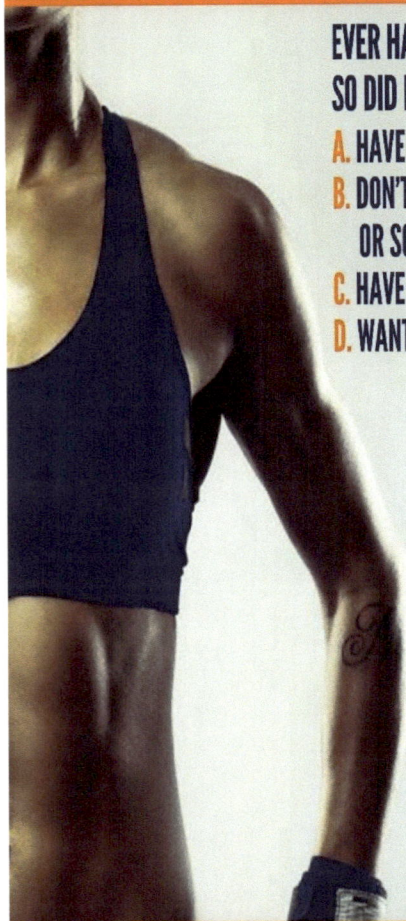

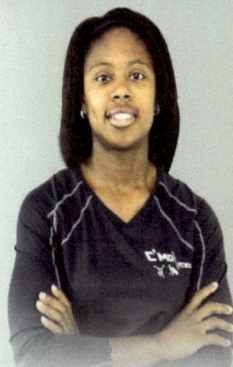

www.ingramcontent.com/pod-product-compliance
Lightning Source LLC
Chambersburg PA
CBHW041303290326
41931CB00032B/33